HIGH and DRY

All about wees, poos and bedwetting

MEG BAMBER
Child Health Nurse

Illustrations BEN RICHARDSON

INTRODUCTION

Hello, my name is Meg.

Welcome to my little book about wees, poos and bedwetting.

For over 30 years I have worked as a Child Health Nurse in Tasmania and for the past 12 years I have proudly been part of a team of Child Health Nurses running Wetaway. This is a program for children aged 5–18 years who are bedwetting and want to be dry at night.

The program is immensely popular and successful, but sadly the nurses are unable to see all the children and families that need help.

Some children have basic bedwetting, and others have problems that need a referral to a specialist Doctor or Physiotherapist.

Sometimes it is a long and frustrating wait to finally get to the Paediatrician (Children's Doctor) then to be asked, "Why are you here?" and sent back to the GP or told, "You just need the alarm [to treat bedwetting]." How disappointing!

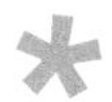

"Bedwetting is such a common problem of childhood, and yet it has lacked a really clear, friendly guide for any parent to use. Meaghan brings years of experience, and a gentle no-fuss approach that has helped hundreds of families."

Steve Biddulph, author of *Complete Secrets of Happy Children, Raising Boys, Raising Girls, 10 Things Girls Need Most* and *The New Manhood*

"Anyone lucky enough to see Meg will know that she affirms everyone in her care, explains what to do in understandable terms and motivates the kids. Meg has a very large body of knowledge and has transferred this into this beautiful new book. How lucky my son has been to see her in person. As a parent, I couldn't recommend this book more highly."

Fiona Scott, mother of an 8-year-old son

"I would like to recommend this easy to read guide which is full of information and encouragement for families struggling with night time wetting."

Hazel Wardlaw, retired family and Child Health Nurse

"Meg's book is full of clear tips and information. It has just enough detail to make it useful and not too much so it becomes overwhelming! I often have children in my classes who have difficulties with using the toilet at school. It's great to have a book I can share with parents, as well as a section specifically for teachers and schools."

Kim Waldron, Special Educator

"An awesome book to help those annoying toileting issues.
Good information for families by the lovely Meg."

Cindy, Child Health Nurse and mother of 11-year-old Lochie

"I loved this little book. It was so easy to read and provides a great resource of practical suggestions for addressing bedwetting in children. A topic that is often hidden, has been brought out in the open in an honest and completely natural manner."

Robyn Sheppard, Physiotherapist APAM

Community programs for bedwetting children are hard to find. Ask first at your local Community Health Centre, your Child Health Nurse, a Continence Nurse, your GP or at a Children's Hospital.

If you live far from health services you can still use an alarm for the bedwetting, and follow the ideas that are in this book.

A special thanks to all the children and their families who have been brave enough to talk about their bedwetting worries and were willing to make some changes.

However, with a thorough GP check, the help of a well-trained Nurse and lots of good information and support, most children will have less wee and poo problems and about 1 in 5 children will become dry at night. Also, children using the alarm will have more success with becoming dry and staying dry.

I am passionate and excited to keep helping children and their families be well and happy.

Please keep reading!

I hope that this book answers your questions about wees, poos and bedwetting. The ideas suggested may reduce some of the problems and will certainly help your child to be ready to see the GP or Nurse.

Very best wishes!

Meg Bamber

Child Health Nurse

HERE ARE 3 STORIES*

ABOUT WEE, POO AND BEDWETTING. DO THEY SOUND FAMILIAR?

wee

A WEE STORY

Amy is 5. She loves school, dancing and anything pink. She is dry at night, and uses the toilet at school – a lot! In fact, she is always wanting to do a wee. She is 'bursting' to go, runs to the toilet, does a quick wee and is keen to get back to class. Sometimes she leaks wee on the way to the toilet, or after doing a wee. She takes spare undies to school, but is shy to ask for help. She has 6 drinks a day, is happy and healthy and sleeps well.

Amy may need to see the GP to check for any poo (bowel) or wee (bladder) problems. (Constipation can cause bladder problems). She may need some prescription medicine from the GP to settle a 'twitchy' bladder. When the bladder muscle is calm, it can get stronger, hold the wee longer and hold bigger wees. Amy may need help from her nurse to have better toilet habits (sitting, wiping and emptying the bladder properly).

Names have been changed in these stories

poo

A POO STORY

Frank is 9. He does not like exercise, but he does love reading and building amazing things with Lego. He does not have any brothers or sisters – he has a goldfish called Midas. Frank loves to eat sausages and potato, but doesn't eat any other vegetable or fruit. Frank does a hard poo every 3 or 4 days and farts a lot! He often has 'skid marks' in his undies. He does not wet the bed, but has damp pyjama pants at night, and wakes up to use the toilet.

Frank may be constipated (full of hard poo). He needs to see his GP (Doctor) for a check-up and a plan to use laxatives (medicine to make the poo soft). He will probably need some help to have better habits: drink more water, eat a mix of healthy foods and have more exercise (to strengthen his tummy muscles).

A BEDWETTING STORY

Johnno is 7 and wets the bed every night. He sleeps really deeply and doesn't wake up to anything! His parents have tried stopping his drinks at 5pm. They also tried 'lifting' him from sleep to use the toilet at 10:30pm on their way to bed. Nothing works. It's hard to get ready to leave on time in the morning as his bed needs changing and Johnno needs to have a shower (so that he doesn't smell of wee). He is busy with friends at school, and forgets to drink. He hates using the school toilet.

Let's book Johnno an appointment with his GP (Doctor) for a general check-up and a nurse appointment for lots of information and support around Healthy Habits: drinking more water at school, using the school toilet when he needs to and having regular bedtimes. His parents may be asked to stop 'lifting' him at night. Johnno may like to try using the bedwetting alarm when he is ready.

bedwetting

Pesky business, this bedwetting, so let's start today with some ideas that will help your child/teenager to have more dry beds (and might also help with some daytime wee/poo problems).

There is information on **HEALTHY HABITS**, lots about wee and poo, when it is time to get help, who is out there that can help, what you can be doing to **get ready** for the first visit to the Nurse or Doctor, what a **bedwetting alarm** is, how to be successful if you use an alarm, when you might need extra **help**, great **books** to read and **websites** for more information and **charts** to print.

Is your child **over 5 years** old, **wets** the bed **most nights**, **wants to be dry at night** and is willing to help?

Time to have a good look at **Healthy Habits**
– perhaps for the whole family!

healthy habits

HEALTHY HABITS

WHAT ARE THESE?

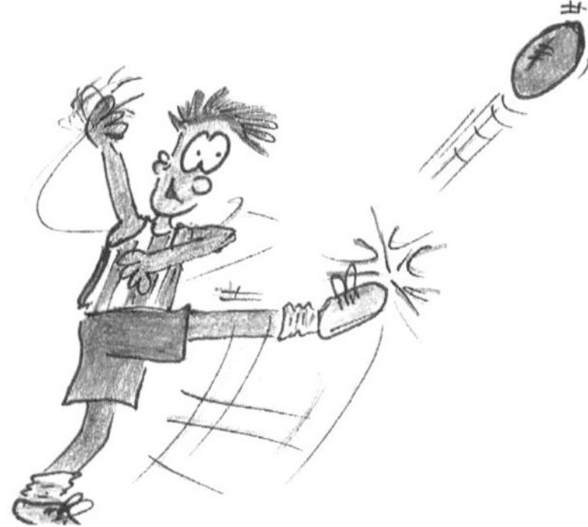

Drinks **6 CUPFULS** of drink **every day**, more on a hot/sports day. Mostly water, some milk.

Food **NATURAL** (unprocessed) foods for **most** meals and snacks.

Sleep Enough good/deep sleep so that you **wake up fresh** and ready to start the day.

Wee About **6–8** pale wees a day.

Poo A sausage-shaped brown poo that **comes out easily** – somewhere between 3 poos a day, and a poo every 3 days.

Exercise **LOTS**, every day!

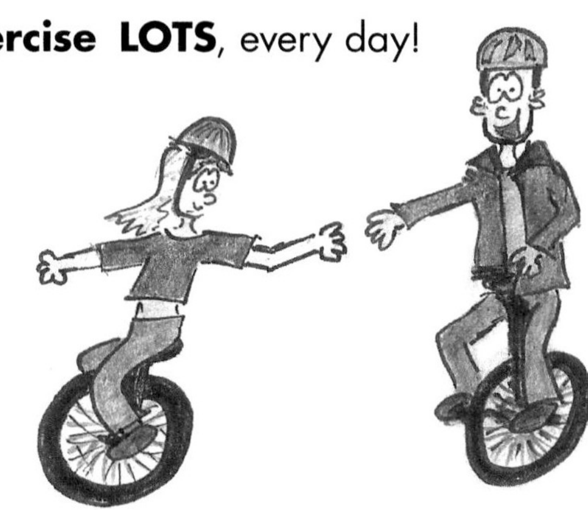

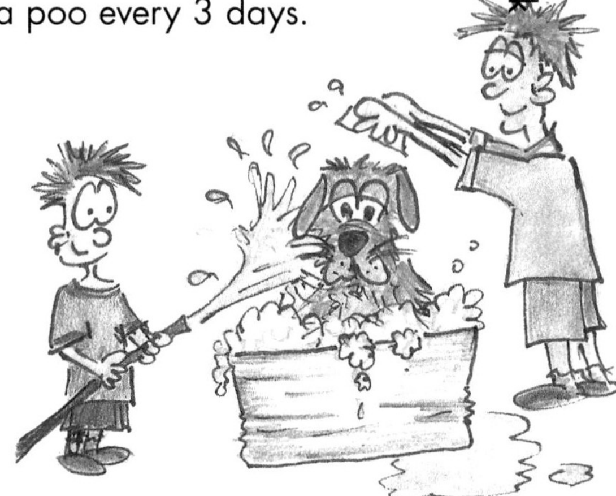

drinks

DRINKS

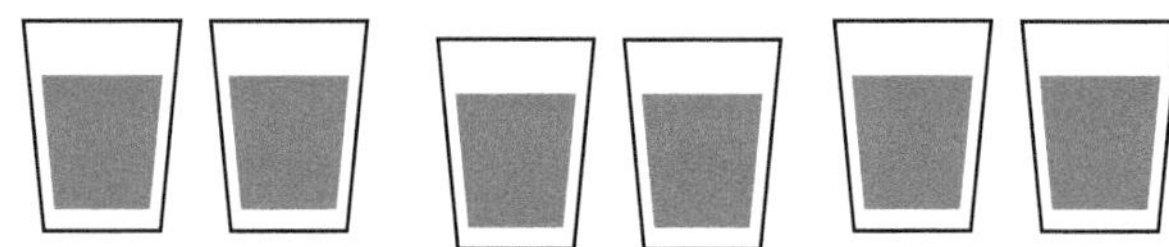

Having enough to drink each day helps you to have a **happy** and **healthy body**, especially your **brain, bladder** (wee) and **bowel** (poo).

THE WHOLE FAMILY COULD TRY THIS

Start your day with **2** drinks **every** day.

Each drink is a **cupful**.

Milk on your cereal counts, and have one extra drink.

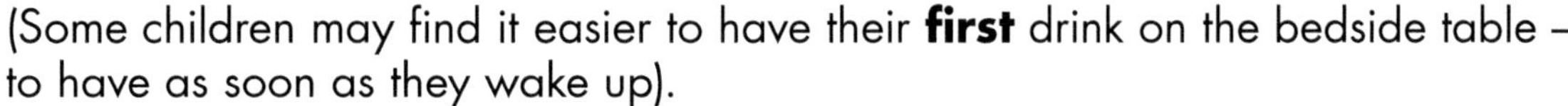

(Some children may find it easier to have their **first** drink on the bedside table – to have as soon as they wake up).

Have another **cupful** at **morning tea**, **lunch**, **afternoon tea** and **dinner**.

6 cupfuls every day. Mostly water, some milk.

Big **cupfuls** (about 300ml) for big people, smaller **cupfuls** (about 150ml) for smaller people.

No more slurps or mouthfuls.

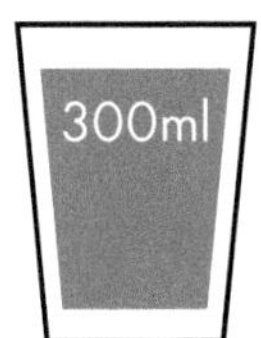

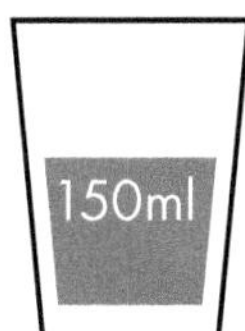

Also try Fruit or herb tea, decaffeinated tea, soy, almond or other milk, milkshakes, homemade fruit & vegetable juice, soup, watermelon, grapes, cucumber & lettuce.

Do choose drinks that are **less sugary**.

drinks

WHO (World Health Organisation) advise having **no more** than

6 teaspoons of sugar each day – for an adult!

That is a **total** of 6 teaspoons of sugar in your drinks **and** your food.

The chart shows how much sugar is in **one** glass of drink of **250ml**.

Please note Store-bought drinks are mostly **375–600ml** or more, so can contain **much more** sugar than a single cup of 250ml.

How much sugar is your child having each day?

More information at www.who.int (nutrition) and www1.health.gov.au

There is a **Drink Chart** to copy and use is at the back of this book.
It may help your child (and you) get used to drinking in cupfuls.

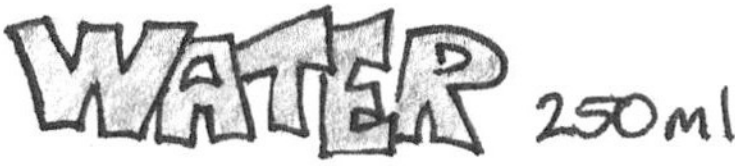

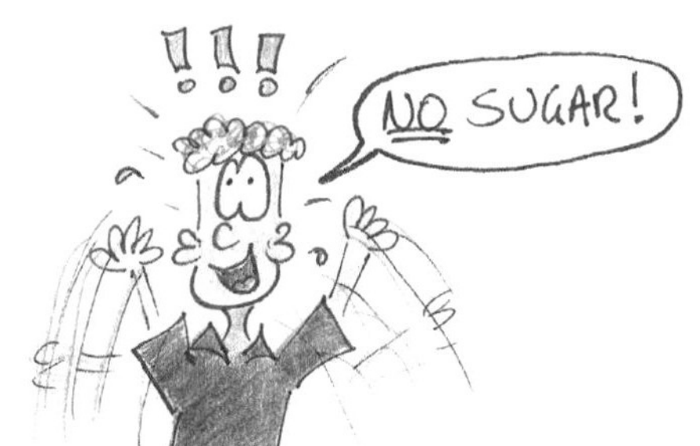

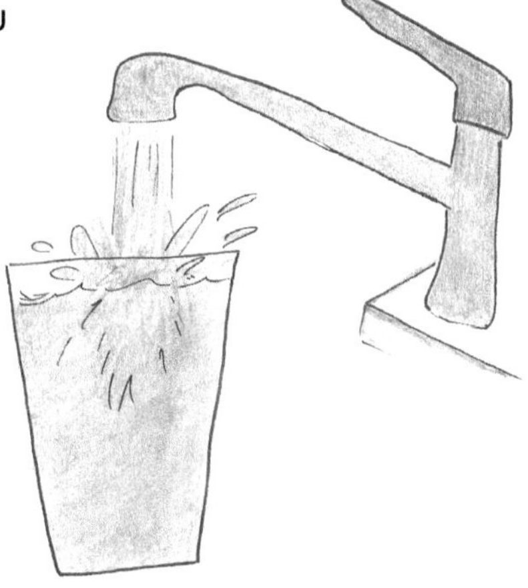

drinks

MILK 250ml

JUST A TINY
BIT OF SUGAR

SPORTS DRINKS 250ml

5 TEASPOONS
OF SUGAR!!!

FLAVOURED
MILK 250ml
3 TEASPOONS
OF SUGAR!!
MILK

250ml FRUIT JUICE
AND
250ml FIZZY DRINKS
6 TEASPOONS OF
SUGAR!!!!

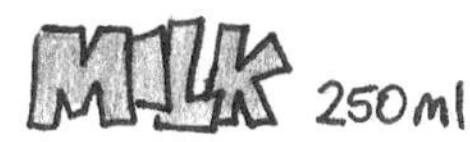

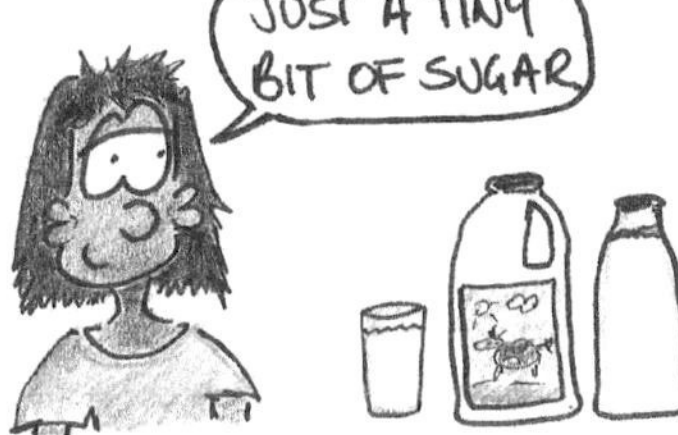

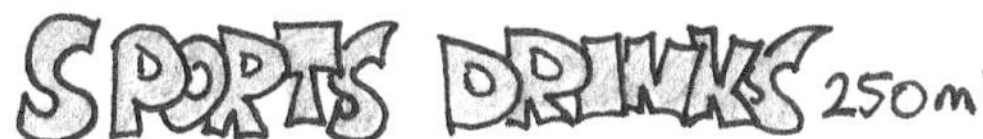

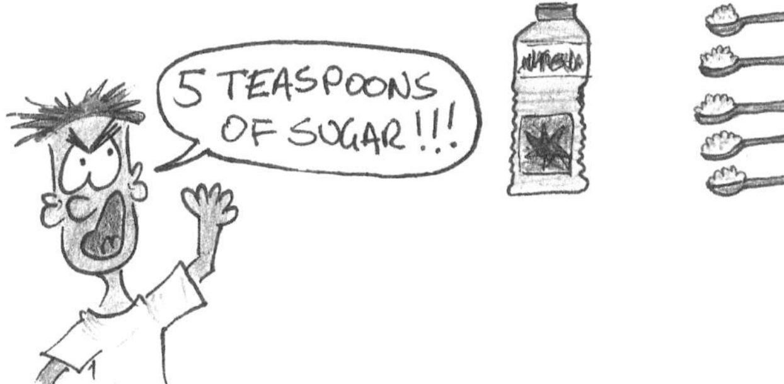

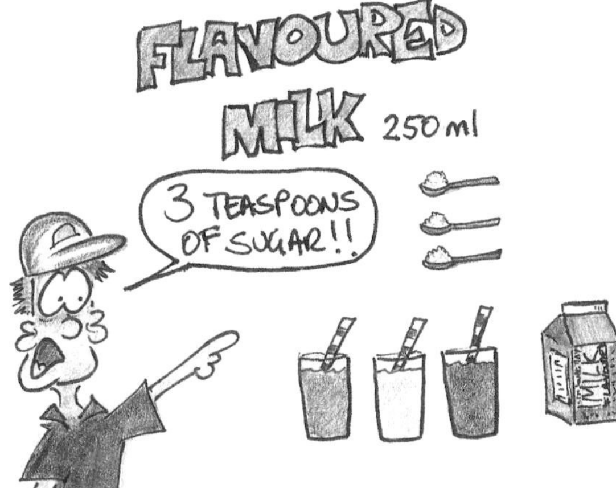

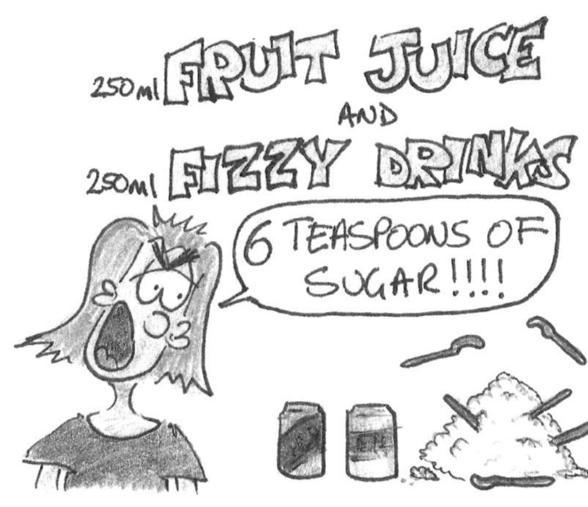

drinks

Do not stop your child having a drink in the evening, or whenever they are thirsty, as this will **not** 'fix' the bedwetting, and might cause other health problems.
If your child has **not been drinking well** for a long time, they might not have the feeling of thirst anymore, as the body becomes used to having less.

Your child may need **extra help** to learn again how to drink well.
Please try using the **Drinks Chart** (at the back of this book) and ask your GP, Child Health Nurse or Community Health Nurse if you need more support.

Is your child **always thirsty**, or seems to drink lots and lots?
Is there are family history of Diabetes?
Please see the **GP**.

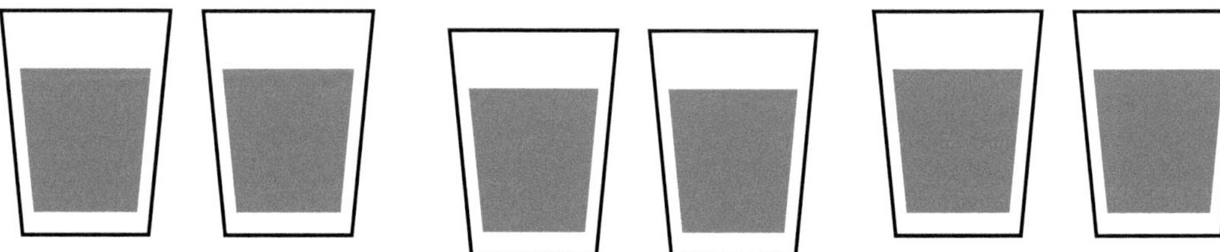

drinks

If your child needs **help** to have bigger drinks:

Week 1 Start with an easy size of perhaps 100mls for **each** of the **6** drinks a day.

Week 2 Make **each** drink size **120ml**, and continue to **increase slowly**, week by week, until your child is easily having bigger drinks.

Aim for a drink size of **150ml**, each drink, for a **small** child; perhaps **300ml** for each drink for a **teenager**.

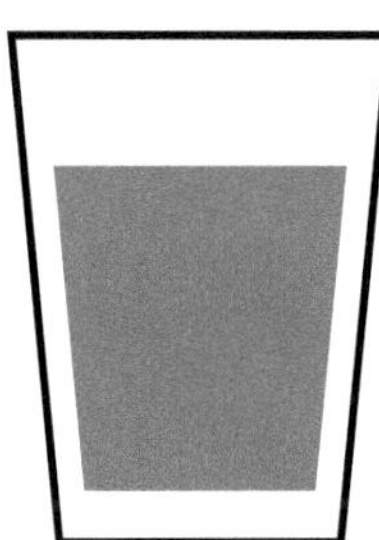

If your child finds it hard to **drink well at school**, have a chat together at the end of each day.

It may be helpful to copy and use the **Drinks Chart** at the end of this book.

Talk about how important it is to have **lots of drinks** each day – to keep our **bodies healthy**, and to have more **dry beds**.

Start again the next day with the drinking plan: **6–8 cupfuls** each day.

food

FOOD

Have some foods from **each different** food group **every** day for growth, repair of your body and ongoing good health.

VEGETABLES & SOME **FRUIT**

for **getting better** after being sick, and to help you **stay well**

Have **lots** every day – enjoy as many different colours and shapes as possible – for extra goodness and fun!

CALCIUM-RICH FOODS for strong teeth and bones

Low-fat milk, low-fat cheese and yoghurt; soy, almond, oat or rice milk that is labelled calcium enriched; canned salmon (with bones), pilchards, sardines with bones; tofu, soybeans, tahini paste, chick peas.

IRON-RICH FOODS for healthy blood and body, and to protect against infection

Liver and kidneys, red meat, chicken, fish, eggs and tofu.

PROTEIN-RICH FOODS for growth, strength and body repair

Fish, chicken, red meat, tempeh, tofu, oats cooked in milk, low-fat milk, low-fat cheese, eggs, baked beans, peanuts, Greek-style yoghurt.

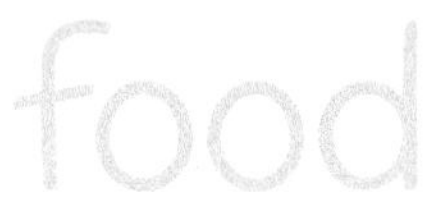

OTHER PROTEIN-RICH FOODS
Mix together **any 2** of these:

Seeds, nuts, grains and legumes. Try lentils and rice, peas and pasta, peanut butter on multigrain bread, homemade muesli, muesli bars, protein balls.

FOR VERY ACTIVE/BUSY/HUNGRY CHILDREN have some **protein-rich** food for **each** snack or meal.

EVERY SNACK IS IMPORTANT:
Try **homemade** popcorn, muesli bars, energy balls, pikelets, savoury muffins, pumpkin scones and cheese, corn fritters, hommus with crackers and veggie sticks, small meatballs/rissoles, homemade chicken nuggets, boiled eggs, toast and nut/seed butter, fruit pieces with plain yogurt and toasted coconut, dried fruit and nuts.

HAVE MORE **NATURAL** (UNPROCESSED) FOOD AT **EACH MEAL**:
Try having porridge for breakfast instead of packet cereal.
Swap white rice to brown rice and white bread to rye or multigrain.
Leave the **skins on** fruit and vegetables whenever possible.

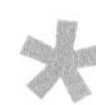

For more information see: www.eatforhealth.gov.au (food plate) and www.heartfoundation.org.au for more snack ideas and recipes.

unhealthy

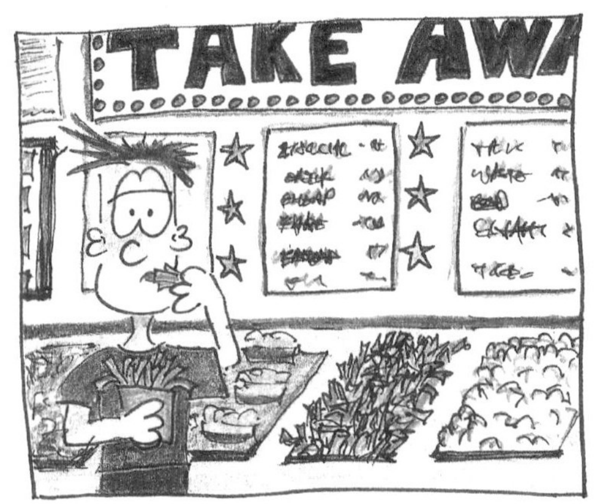

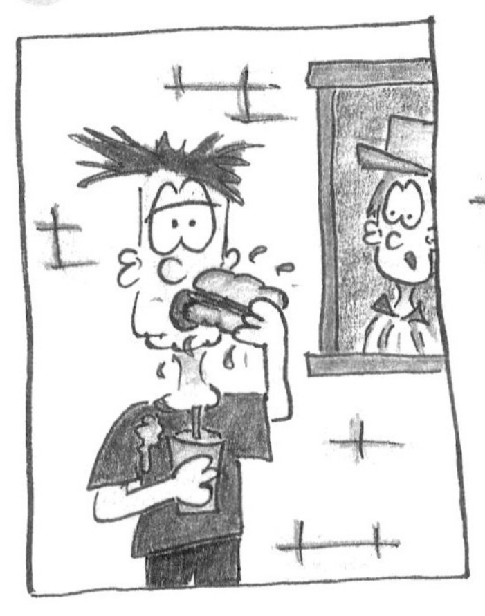

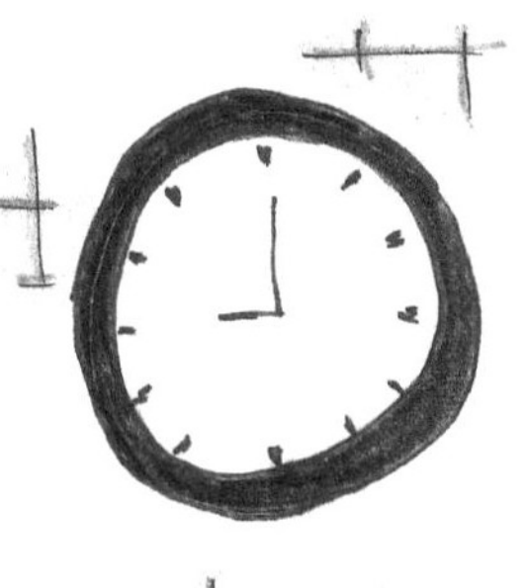

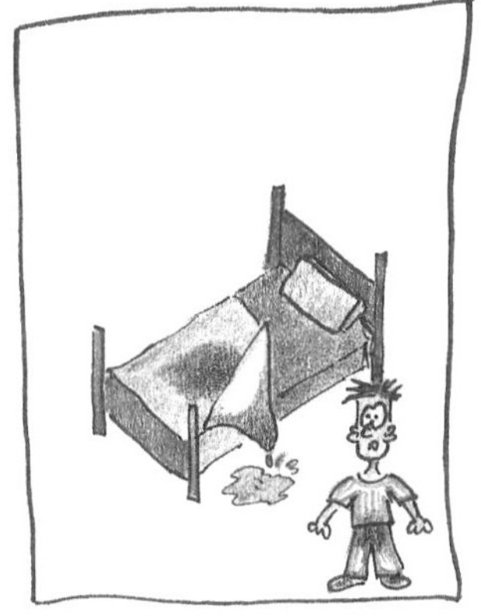

SUGARY + SALTY = MORE WET BEDS

SUGARY AND SALTY FOOD AND DRINKS LEAD TO MORE ***WET*** *BEDS*

healthy

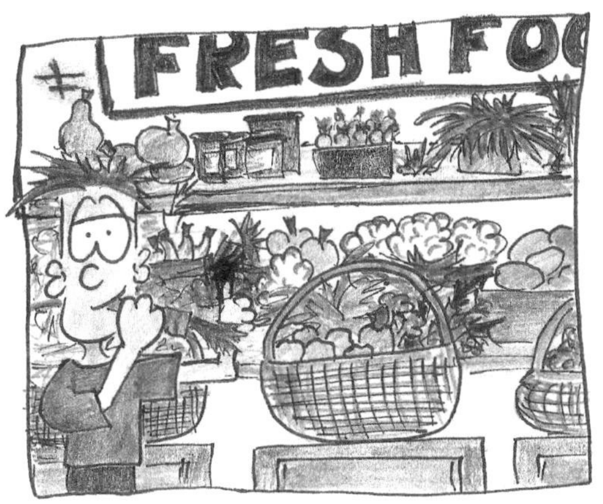

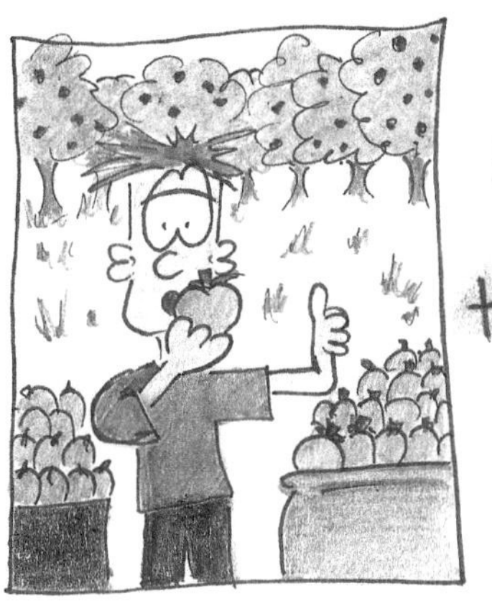

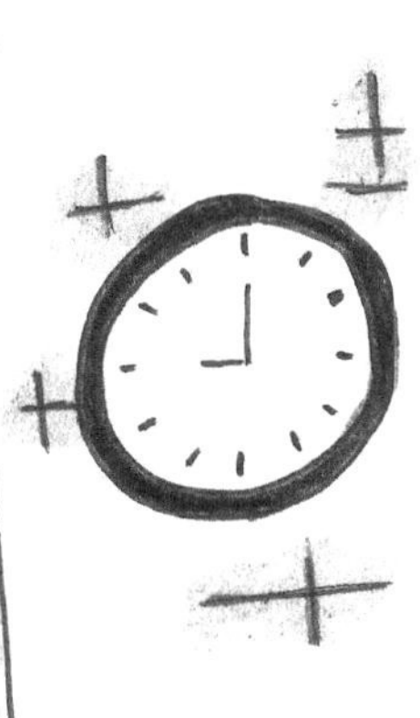

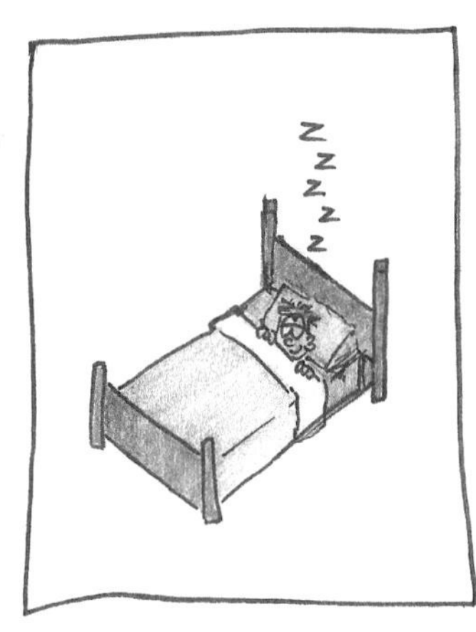

HEALTHY FOOD + HEALTHY DRINKS = MORE DRY BEDS

HEALTHY FOOD AND DRINKS LEAD TO MORE **DRY** *BEDS*

sleep

SLEEP

SLEEPING WELL

Getting **enough sleep** means we wake up '**fresh** and **ready**' for the day and helps the **brain** to 'hear' better the **wee and poo messages**.

We have several **sleep cycles** each night. Each sleep cycle is about 90 minutes long, and goes from light to deep sleep.

DURING **LIGHT SLEEP**

We notice if something has changed: like the cat jumping onto the bed, it has started to rain, your arm has gone to sleep, or you need to do a wee. In light sleep the brain can 'hear' the body messages more easily.

At Primary School age, it is **normal** for your child to **sleep deeply** and not wake up to noise and wet beds.

DURING **DEEP SLEEP** (and Primary School children need lots of this) the body makes the **Growth Hormone** – something that is very important and helps your child to grow **bigger** and **stronger**.

As your child grows older, their brain will 'hear' more loudly the wee messages while asleep. Eventually they will wake to use the toilet.

sleep

TO HAVE BETTER SLEEP

Help your child to go to bed at the **same time** each night.

No screen time for **1 hour** before bed – this means **no** computers, iPads,television or mobile phones (parents too!).

(The light coming from these gadgets 'wakes up' the brain).

Get out the board games, pack of cards, jigsaw puzzles, and paper books!

Read together, tell stories, look at family photos.

IF YOUR CHILD SLEEPS 'HOT'

TRY A warm (not hot!) shower for your child at bedtime.

Summer pyjamas or sleep bare.

Wipe down the body with a little cornflour. (Cornflour can feel soothing and absorbs sweat).

Less bedcovers at bedtime – you could place another blanket over your child when you are on your way to bed.

IF YOUR CHILD IS COLD AT NIGHT

TRY A very warm shower for your child at bedtime.

Warm pyjamas and a singlet underneath, maybe bedsocks.

An extra blanket over your child.

Do you need to warm the bedroom?

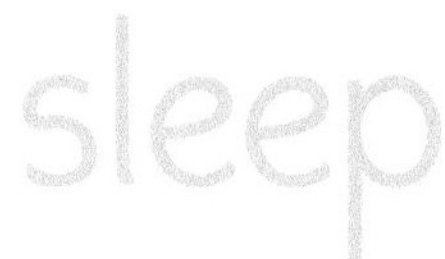

IF YOUR CHILD NEEDS TO BE WOKEN IN THE MORNING, or is hard to wake up, he/she may need to go to bed earlier.

MAKE CHANGES SLOWLY

Week 1 Try bringing bedtime 10 minutes earlier: eg 7:20 pm instead of 7:30 pm.

Week 2: Change bedtime again by another 10 minutes: eg 7:10 pm instead of 7:20 pm.

Do this a few times, until the child **wakes easily** in the morning, in time to get ready for school.

DOES YOUR CHILD HAVE TROUBLE GOING TO SLEEP, OR STAYING ASLEEP?

Does your child sleepwalk, sleeptalk, snore, grind teeth, have restless legs, have nightmares or night terrors?

Is there a **family history** of any sleep problems, or anxiety? If so, please have a chat with your **GP** or friendly Pharmacist.

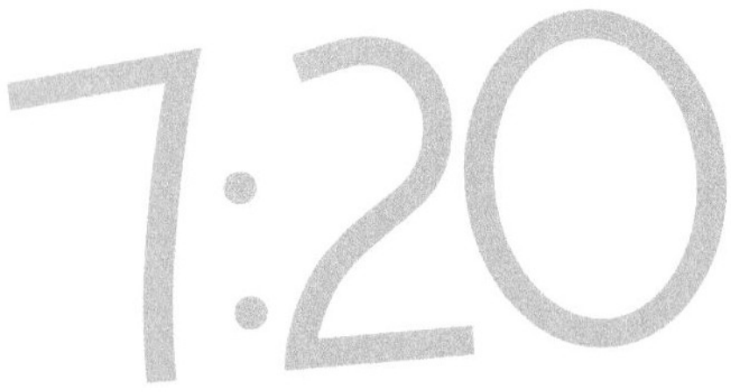

things to try

SOME THINGS TO TRY

- Gentle **music**.
- **Read** to your child.
- Keep your child **company** – sit in a comfy chair near your child, read your favourite book while your child goes to sleep.
- Some children find a **back/foot rub** soothing, also hair brushing/stroking.
- A small cup of **warm milk** with a little honey, at bedtime.
- Listen to the '**Smiling Mind**' app.
- **Yoga** breathing and/or yoga stretches – great for mums and dads too!
- A 'weighted' or **heavy blanket**.
- **Natural therapies**, Homeopathy, Aromatherapy.
- **Acupressure**/Acupuncture.
- **Osteopathy**.
- Trial of Melatonin medicine – talk to the **GP**.

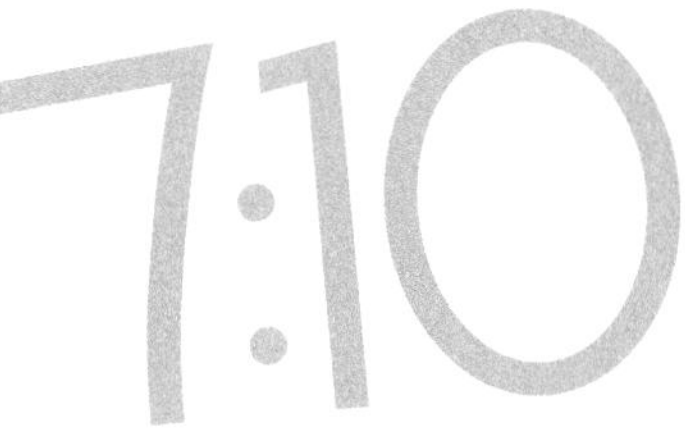

wees

WEES

A **HEALTHY WEE** is **pale**, not smelly, comes out in a **strong**, **steady stream** and is about **150ml** or more. (Your child will need to wee into a container. Pour the wee into a laundry jug with measures on it, and check the wee size before flushing the wee down the toilet).

Whenever you get/feel a **wee** or (**poo message**), **stop** what you are doing, and **go to the toilet**!

Having **good toilet habits** and **drinking in cupfuls** will help the bladder to hold **bigger** wees and send '**louder**' messages to the brain.

Doing this in the daytime helps the brain to remember that a wee or poo message means **use the toilet**! and will help your child later on to **wake at night** to use the toilet.

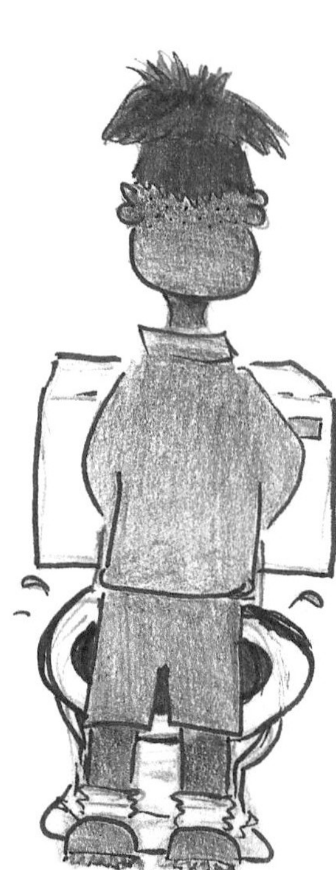

wees

Most people do about **6-8** wees a day.

After **having a cupful** of water, it takes **20–30 minutes** for the bladder to fill.

As the **bladder fills**, the **muscle** around the bladder **twitches**, sending a **message** up the spine to the **brain**.

The brain '**hears**' the message, and sends a message back down the **spine**, to the bladder, telling you to **stop** what you are doing, and **go to the toilet**.

Think of your spine like a Super Highway, going from Hobart to Launceston! (If you live in Tasmania).

We want the messages going up and down to be **fast**, **loud** and **clear**!

THINGS THAT CAN UPSET THE BLADDER AND MAKE IT 'TWITCHY'
Try to have less of these:

- Sugary and salty foods
- Sugary drinks, fizzy and sports drinks
- Juice from a carton
- Artificial colours and flavours (in many foods and drinks).

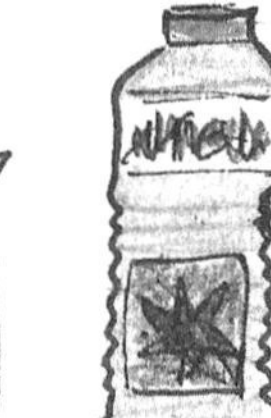

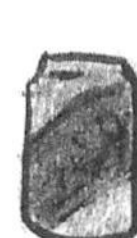

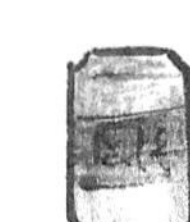

DO HAVE

- Lots of water and some milk. About **6–8 cupfuls** every day.

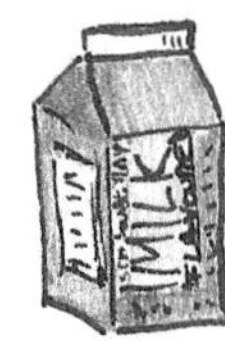

things to try

SOME THINGS TO TRY

TO HELP YOUR CHILD GET TO THE TOILET/BE DRY AT NIGHT

Encourage your child to **do a wee** as they **start** to get ready for bed, and another wee **just before** lights out

Move your child to the **bottom bunk** (easier/faster to get to the toilet!)

Is the **toilet** far from the child's bedroom? You could try putting a bucket/potty in the bedroom for the child to wee into.

Is there **enough light** at night? Ask your child. You could make a 'runway' of nightlights from the bedroom to the toilet or put a torch under the child's pillow.

Is the **floor cold**? Put slippers at the bedside.

Have a 'furry friend' ready as **company** for your child.

Let your child know that it is OK if they **call you** at night for some help.

Whenever your child **wakes during the night** please help them to get up and use the toilet.

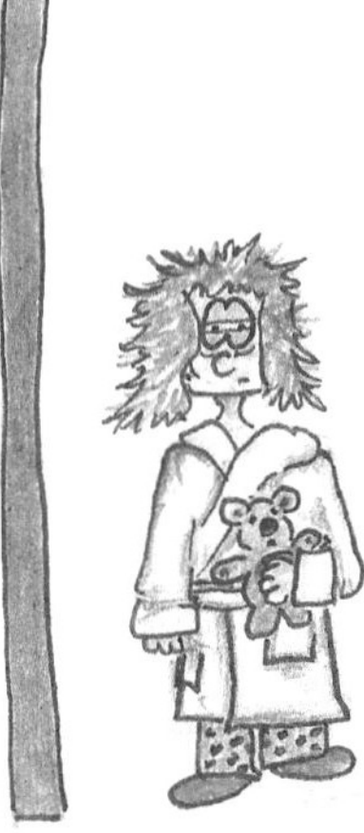

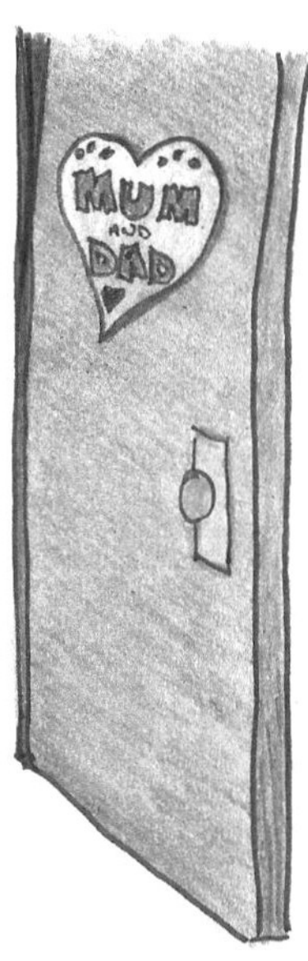

HERE IS

A FAMILY WEE CHALLENGE

wee challenge

When the family gets back home **everyone go to the toilet and do a wee.**

Everyone have a cupful of drink, then wait to see who gets the **'wee message' first** (about 20–30 minutes).

'Listen' to the wee message and go and do a wee in the toilet.

Are you brave enough to measure your wee? Whose is biggest?

Is it more than 150ml? (You will need to wee into a container to measure the wee). 150ml or more is a healthy wee size for a small child.

You may find it useful to use the **Wee Chart** (find one at the back of this book) and measure wees for a few days – this will show how the bladder is behaving and if your child needs help.

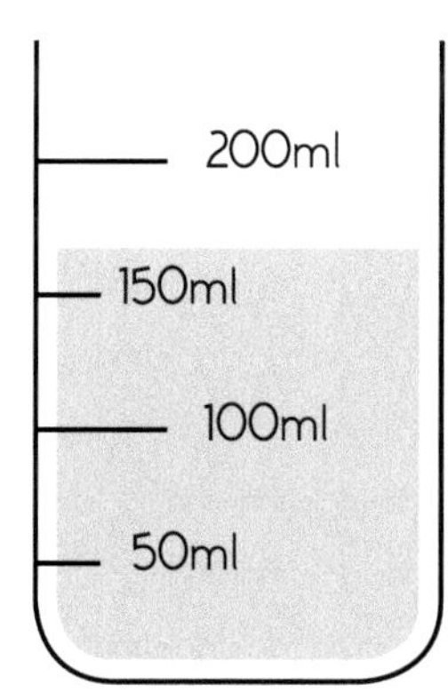

wee activity

A WEE ACTIVITY

When your child has done a few wee measures (using the **wee chart** at the back of this book), look together to find the **smallest** wee and the **biggest** wee eg 40ml and 180ml.

Take a **balloon** to the kitchen, find a **measuring jug** and a small **funnel**.

Measure the amount of the **smallest** wee (eg 40ml) as tap water into the jug.

Place the funnel into the balloon opening, and pour in the water.

Then you can both see **the size of the bladder** holding a **small wee**.

Tip the water out, and again using tap water, measure the **biggest** amount (eg 180ml) into the jug and pour this bigger amount into the balloon.

Now you can both see how much **bigger** the bladder is when holding a **bigger wee**!

This will help your child to understand what is happening to the bladder and the difference between a small wee and a big wee.

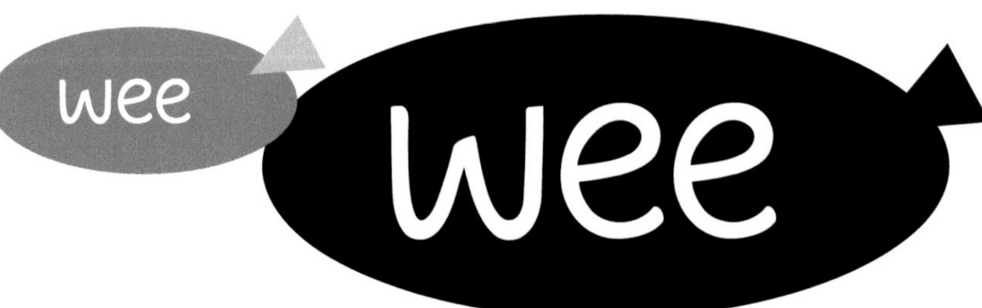

the toilet

USING THE TOILET

... AND STOPPING THE WEE OR POO ACCIDENTS

Go to the toilet whenever you get the **wee** (or **poo**) **message**.
Slow down the visit to the toilet so that the **bladder** has time to **fully empty**.

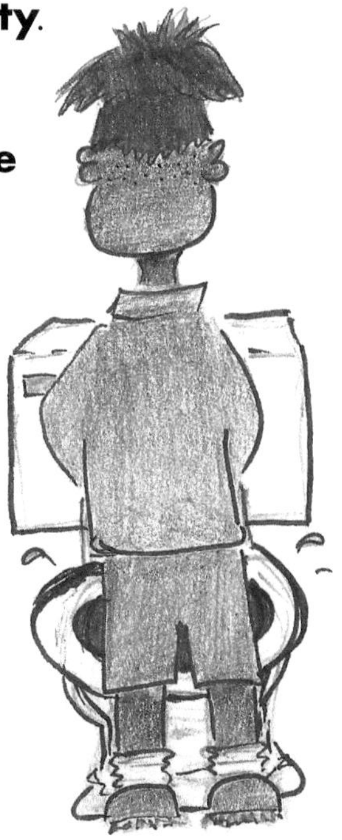

BOYS DO THIS **Stand and wee** and when you feel finished **wriggle** your hips for a few seconds, then **finish your wee** (a bit more wee will probably come out).

GIRLS DO THIS **Sit and wee** and when you feel finished stand and **wriggle** your hips for a few seconds, then **sit** again and **finish your wee** (a bit more wee will probably come out).

BOYS AND GIRLS **After a poo**
go back to the toilet to **do a wee** (empty the bladder) again about 20 minutes **after** doing a poo.

* *These things may help to stop any leaky business/accidents!*

IF YOUR CHILD 'HOLDS ON' TO THE WEE

Over time, the **bladder muscle** can **stretch** (like loose elastic) and is no longer sending a strong or 'loud' message to the **brain**.

wees

Try having **regular visits** to the toilet: about every **2–3 hours**.

The bladder muscle will get **stronger**, the bladder will return to a **normal size** and the 'wee' messages will be '**loud and clear'** again.

Your child may need some **help** from a Physio with this.

PRACTISE THIS AT HOME

Remind your child to go to the toilet about every **2–3** hours.
Using a friendly voice tell them, "**It's time to go to the toilet**", rather than asking them "Would you like to go?"
Try using the stove timer, or a phone alarm, to help with the reminders.

brrrrnnnggg! It's time to go

Please DO NOT do any bladder or **pelvic floor exercises** until you have checked with a **Physio**.

hygiene

Sometimes children get a **wee** (urine) **infection** (more often with girls).

To help stop this happening encourage girls to wipe with toilet paper from '**front to back**' after using the toilet.

It may be helpful to **clean the bottom after** doing a **poo** and **before** having **a bath**. This gets rid of poo germs.

Wipe bottoms gently with a wet, soapy cloth.
Wipe the soap off and wipe dry.
Place the cloth straight into the washing machine.

Or wipe bottoms clean with a little bit of sorbolene cream on toilet paper.
Sorbolene cream is in the supermarket in a pump pack.

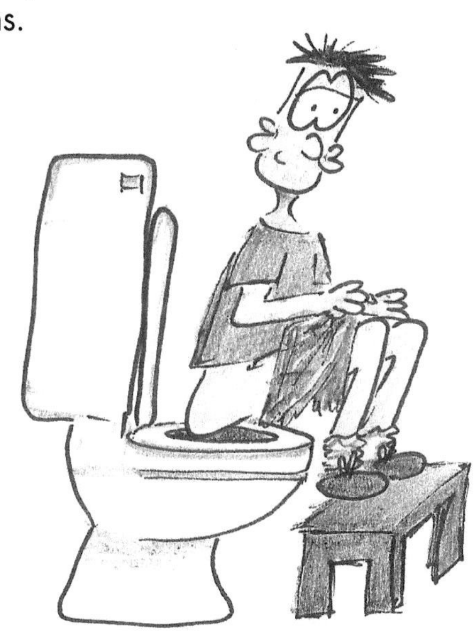

WHAT IS TOO MUCH WEE (FREQUENCY/URGENCY)**?**

If your child seems to be doing **lots and lots** of small wees,
do the **Wee** (measuring) **Chart** for **a few days**,
as the information will help the Nurse, a GP or Physio.

They will check the **wee sizes**, and **how many** wees each day.

Sometimes the bladder can be very '**twitchy**', and the 'wee messages' don't stop coming.

The **GP** may prescribe some **medicine** that will help to **calm**/settle the bladder.
This will allow the bladder to be able to **hold** on to **wees**
for **longer**, and to **hold bigger wees**.

Your child may need extra help from a **Physio**
with pelvic floor exercises.
Always check with a Physio first
before doing these!

* *See Wee Chart on page 65*

use the Wee Chart

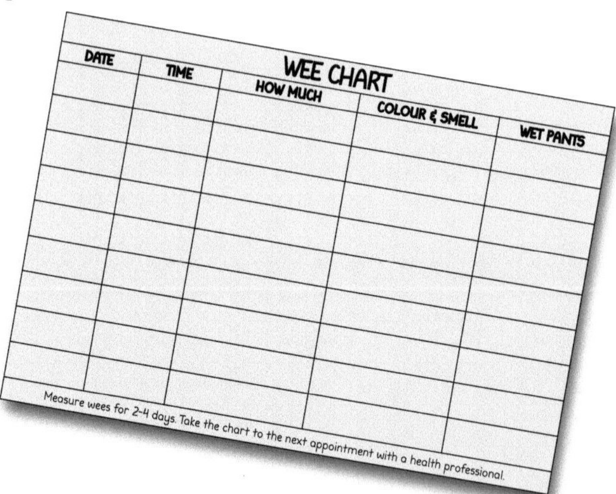

soaked beds

SOAKED BEDS EVERY NIGHT?

Usually the body makes **less wee** when asleep.
It is normal to wake **once** or **twice** a night to do a wee in the toilet – as long as you can go back to sleep!

If your child's nappy, pyjamas and bed are **soaked every night**, there may be a medical problem.
Use the **Wee Chart** at the back of this book to write down the **weight** of the **dry** nappy and pyjama pants before bedtime.

In the morning **weigh** the **soaked** nappy and pyjama pants **and add** the measure of the **first wee** of the day.
(Note: 400ml equals 400 grams).

Do this for at least **7 days**.

If the amount is **always large** (over 400ml), check with the **GP** and take the chart with you.
Sometimes the problem (of making too much wee at night) can be helped by a **prescription medicine** from the **GP**.

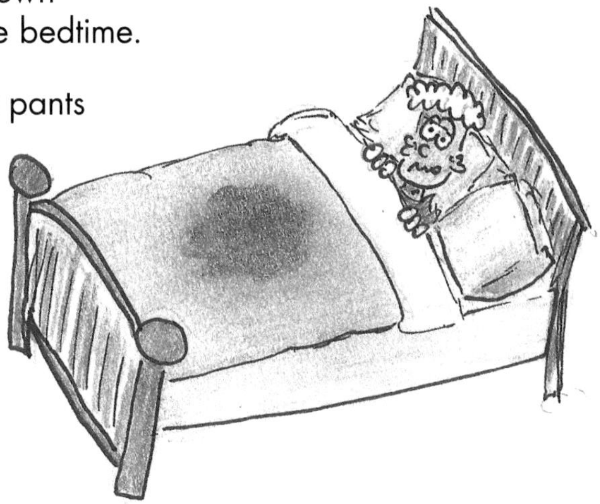

POO poo

A healthy poo is **brown**, **soft and sausage-shaped**, comes out **easily**, without grunting or lots of pushing and takes about **2–5 minutes**.

It is OK to do a poo **every 3 days** or even up to **3 poos a day**.

We usually get the feeling to do a poo about **20** minutes **after** a meal.

SITTING ON THE TOILET, FOR EVERYONE

Good toilet posture helps the poo to come out easily!

Sit with your bottom towards the **back** of the toilet seat.

Your **knees** need to be **higher** than your **hips**. (You may need to keep a **box** or **small stool** in the toilet room to put under your feet).

Keep your **feet flat** on the stool or box.

Send a message to the tummy to '**relax**' and let the poo '**fall**' **out**.

Small children may be able to **squat** on the toilet seat with feet flat (like doing a poo when you are camping/in the bush).

Stay nearby to keep them safe.

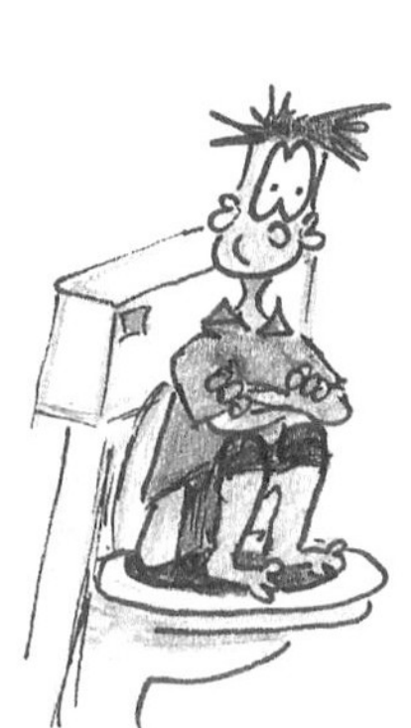

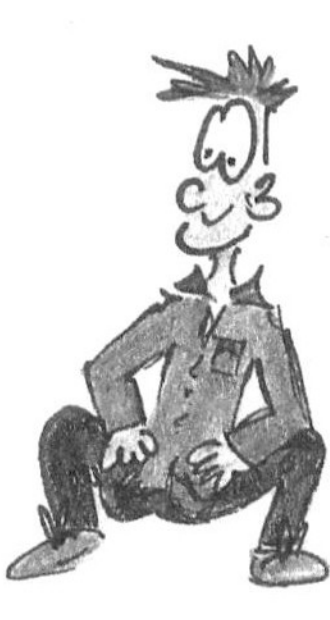

poo

REMEMBER
When you get the poo message, **stop** what you are doing, and **go to the toilet**.

IF THE POO IS SLOW TO COME OUT:

When you are **sitting** on the toilet:

Try making **hissing** noises (like a slithery snake) – you will feel your lower tummy tighten.

Perhaps you can **whistle**?

Blow some bubbles (when you are at home).
Some children may need help/reminding to sit on the toilet for **2–5** minutes,
3 times a day **after** meals, until they are doing a poo easily.

POO CHALLENGE

Have everyone in the family **eat some corn** on the cob (or some beetroot or some currants) and ask who can **see the corn** in their poo first!

This may be as fast as **12 hours**, or for a slower gut, up to **3 days**.
Everyone's gut (insides) has a different speed.
The important thing is that the **poo comes out easily**!

CHECK YOUR POO

www.continence.org.au – Bristol Stool Chart.

constipation

CONSTIPATION (HARD POO)

Hard poo, or a **build-up of poo,** can make the child feel **unwell**, have **stomach pains**, or have **bladder** (stores the wee) problems or **bowel** (stores the poo) problems. If the poo is very **slow** to come out, is very **hard** or **hurts** – check again the list of **Healthy Habits** to see if anything needs to change.

Does your child need encouraging to **drink** more, **exercise** more, have **more natural** and less packaged foods? Try more vegetables, fruit, brown rice, oats, beans and lentils. (Leave the skins on the fruit and vegetables where possible).
Perhaps try **Probiotics** (from the pharmacy – to help with a healthy gut).

A **GP** can check for a **build-up of poo** (constipation) in the bowel. They will feel your child's tummy and may order a test if needed (X-ray or ultrasound).
If possible, **before the GP visit**, please fill in the **Poo Chart*** (at the back of this book) and take to your GP.
It will help the GP to help your child.
7 days using the poo chart is good, **14 days** is **better**!

DO NOT WAIT if your child is unwell or in pain!

POO CHART

DATE	TIME	HOW MUCH	COLOUR & TYPE	SOILING

Measure poos for 7-14 days. Take the chart to the next appointment with a health professional.

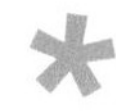

See Poo Chart on page 67

Sometimes a **treatment** (laxative) needs to be used to soften the poo.

If the problem has been there for a long time, the bowel may have stretched.

It may take a few **months** of treatment and special exercises for the bowel to return to normal – get some **help** with this from your **GP** or **Physio**.

Keep going being **kind and patient** with your child – it is frustrating for them too!

soiling

SOILING

Pesky poo in the underpants can be from:

- **Waiting too long** to go to the toilet after getting the poo message,
- Being in a hurry and not **wiping properly** after doing a poo.
- Some poo coming out with a **fart**
  (farts can be a message that it is time to go to the toilet!)
- Sometimes poo can **leak** out around a **build-up of poo** in the bowel – time to get some **help** from the **GP** or **Physio**.

EXERCISE

At least **1 hour** of exercise **every day** –
something that makes you 'huff and puff'.

Strong muscles will help your bladder and bowel to work better.

Riding a bike, scooter or skateboard, playing sports,
dancing, helping in the garden,
or helping with jobs inside the house.
Do you have some grassy hills to walk up and roll down?

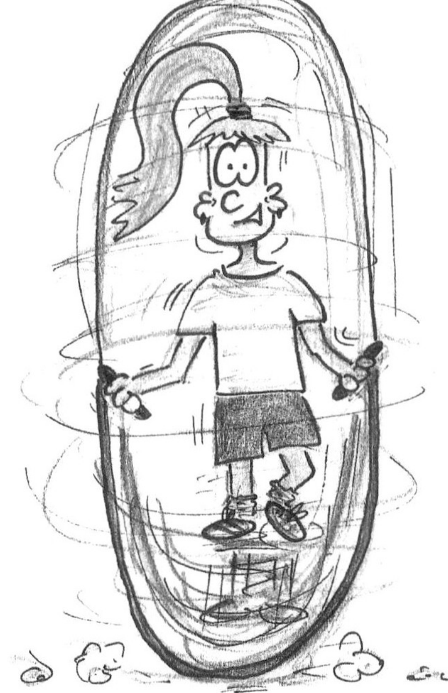

Make a list of **outside games**
and **inside games**
that your child (and you) enjoys.
How about some old favourites:
Hopscotch, skittles, marbles and
building a cubby house!

DOES YOUR CHILD HAVE

WEIRD WEES, PESKY POOS OR FUNKY FARTS?

WHEN TO GO TO THE GP, NURSE OR PHYSIO

- **Anytime that you are worried** about your child's wee or poo (or anything else).
- If the **wee or poo problems do not get better** after trying the **Healthy Habits**.
- If there are any **family problems** with wee, poo, kidney, bladder or bowel.
- If your child does not **'feel'** the wee or poo messages, or does not notice the leaky business/accidents.
- **Anytime** that **you** think that something is **not quite right**.

COMPLETE THE WEE AND POO CHARTS (at the end of this book) and take them with you to the appointment with a Nurse, GP or Physio.

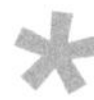

This information will make it easier to work out the problem, and find the best person to help.

school

AT SCHOOL

Is your child **using the school toilets** – for both wee and poo?
Ask them! Some children will only poo in the toilet at home.

Check with the teacher: how do the children ask when they need to use the toilet?
Can your child go whenever they need to?

If possible, it is helpful to have a big **drink 30 minutes before** recess or lunch.
Then the bladder is full and ready to do wees **at recess**.

Often the child is **back in class** after recess **then** needs the toilet.
The teacher may not allow the child to leave the classroom again so soon.

What are the school toilets like – have you had a look?
How far are the school toilets from the classroom? Is this a problem?

A **vibrating watch** may be helpful to remind your child when to use the toilet.
These are available online, or from some pharmacies. (About $80).

Put together a little **zip up bag** with tissues, spare undies & shorts, and anything else that your child may need if they have a wee or poo accident at school. Make sure they know **who** to ask for help and **where** to go to **change** their undies and **freshen up**.

SCHOOL CAMPS, HOLIDAYS AND SLEEPOVERS

Keep things as normal as possible.

Encourage your child to go on outings.

Talk with them about ways to manage the wetting: pull-ups, spare pyjamas and some stick-on absorbent bed mats (in supermarkets, near nappies).

The stick-on bed mats can be used inside a sleeping bag, below your child's bottom. You can also stick a mat inside the bag above your child's hips, as some boys wee up!

Talk to the **GP** about using some **prescription medicine** to help your child to make less wee at night.

Sometimes children stop bedwetting **while away** on a sleepover, camping, travelling on a family holiday or staying at the beach shack.

This is because they **sleep less deeply** when away from home – the bedwetting is not fixed yet!

Wait for **2–3 weeks**, after coming home, to see if the bedwetting starts again.

returning to school

RETURNING TO SCHOOL after holidays can be tricky, as your child may have been drinking enough with you around but forgets to drink well at school.
Keep encouraging 2 drinks at breakfast time.

Make it really easy by having **1** or **2 small drink bottles** already marked with cupfuls (amounts that your child can easily manage).

Encourage your child to **measure a cupful** into their drink bottle the **night before** school.

Mark the bottle here and add a **second** cupful.

The **first** cupful is to have at **recess**, the **second** cupful at **lunchtime**.

If this doesn't work, try having **2** small bottles, with **1 cupful** (1 serve) in **each** bottle. One to have at **recess** and one at **lunchtime**.

If **this** doesn't work encourage: **2 cups** of water **straight after school**, **1 cupful** at **5 pm**, **1** with **dinner** and we are back on track!

Drinking lots late in the day makes a wet bed **more** likely as there isn't enough time for the body to make all the wee that needs to come out.

Well done and keep going!

With **your help and support**, it is easier for your child to remember the Healthy Habits.

information

EXTRA INFORMATION

FOR THE GP, NURSE OR PHYSIO

Are there any **family problems** with **wee**, **bladder** or **kidneys**?

Has your child had any wee (bladder or kidney) infections?

Does your child do **lots of very small wees** every day? (10–20).

Does your child **leak wee** on the way to, or after using, the toilet.

Does your child **leak wee** after jumping, sneezing or coughing?

Does your child seem to **hold** onto the wee for hours, or **cannot hold on** to the wee, or is always 'bursting' to go?

Check '**Using the Toilet'** information first – do any toilet habits need changing?

Is the wee dark, smelly, hurts when it comes out?

Try having an **extra** 2 drinks each day.

See the GP if it hurts to wee, there is no change, or you are worried.

Does the wee come out in dribbles, a sideways squirt, in 'stops and starts' or as a **strong steady stream**?

Please **fill in the Wee and Poo charts**, and **take** them with you to your **appointment** with the Nurse, GP or Physio.

Lots of information makes it **easier** for them to help your child.

information

INFORMATION
FOR TEACHERS, CARERS AND AFTER-SCHOOL CARE

Please **encourage everyone** to have a cupful of water at **recess**, **lunchtime** and at **After-school Care.**

Even better if everyone can have a drink **30 minutes before** a break – this gives the bladder time to fill and be ready to do a wee. (Try it!)

Please encourage the children to use the toilet at recess and at lunchtime, and make it OK for them to go to the toilet at other times as they need.
Some children are happier to use the toilet if a friend can walk with them.

If you notice someone not drinking well, not using the toilet, or having any wee or poo problems, **please tell the parent/carer**, as they may not know this.

Some children need extra help to remember to **drink** and to **use the toilet**, as games and friends are far more interesting!

WHILE YOUR CHILD IS BECOMING DRY

Give them **lots** of **encouragement** and **support**.

You might find it helpful to use a very absorbent **bed mat** (from department stores or medical supply shops) – it will soak up lots of wee. It will take longer to dry but will keep your child **feeling dry** and **comfy** at night. (You may need 2 or 3).

A **polar fleece blanket** is quick to wash and dry. (Put the good doona or blanket away for a while).

Be ready to help your child during the night. Keep using nappies or **pull-ups** if you need to, while **checking** the **Healthy Habits** and **making changes**, or while **waiting** for a bedwetting alarm.

For safety reasons
please DO NOT use an electric blanket
for anyone who wets the bed!

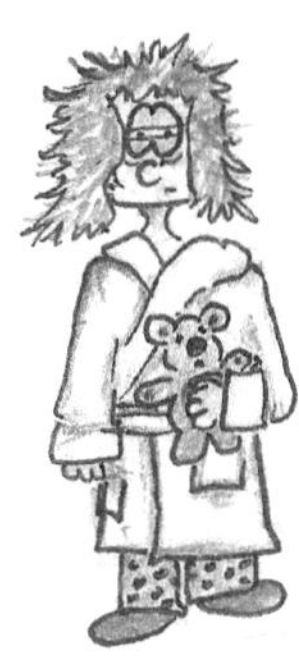

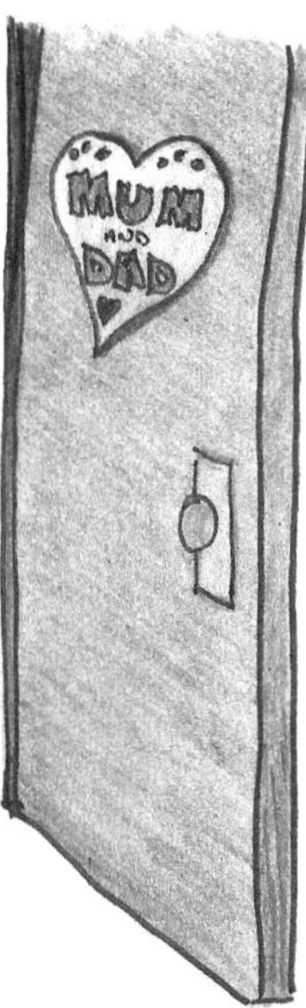

alarms

ALARMS
IS YOUR CHILD READY?

The alarm will be more successful if the child is **over 6** years.

The body is **more mature** at this time, and the **brain** is better at **sending** and **receiving** messages to and from the **bladder**.

Before using the alarm, have you checked the **Healthy Habits** – did you need to make any changes?

Did they work?

beep beep

Has your child had a **check-up** with the **GP**?

Do this **before** using the alarm.

The GP will check your child's **health**, wee or poo problems, past illness and order more checks only if needed (blood, wee or poo check, X-ray or ultrasound).

Did the GP say it is **OK** to try the alarm?

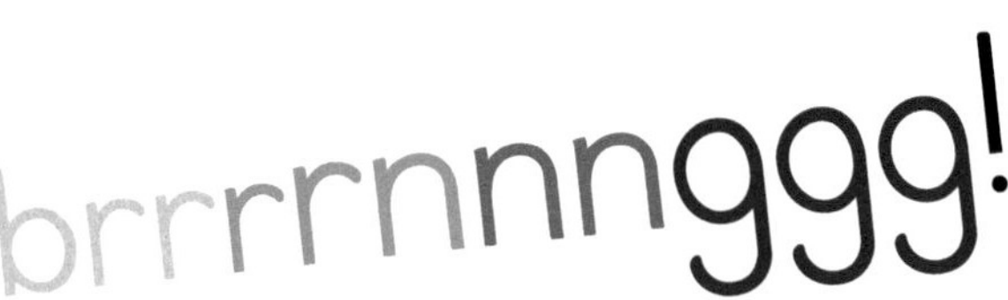

alarms

IS YOUR CHILD ...

- Still **wetting most nights**?
- Drinking better at school? Having **6 cupfuls** a day?
- **Drinking** mostly water and some milk?
- **Eating** mostly **healthy** foods?
- Doing **wees of 150ml** or more?
- Doing a regular and **soft poo**?
- Having plenty of **exercise**?
- **Sleeping** well?
- Is your child **well**, and **ready** to use the alarm?

brr brr

Is it a good time for you?

Do you have a new baby, new house, or are about to go on holidays?
Have there been any other **big changes** in the family (someone passing away or leaving home)?

Are you **happy to help** at night while your child is using the alarm?
Have any **wee or poo problems** been sorted?

alarms

HAS YOUR CHILD ...

TRIED SLEEPING WITHOUT NAPPIES?

If not, before using the alarm, try for up to 5 nights in a row without night nappies to see if your child **wakes to the wetness** or is **more dry** at night.

As your child gets **older** the brain will '**listen**' **better** to wee messages. Just now your child may be wetting the bed and not waking.

Signs of improvement with or without the alarm

1. Your child will wake **after** wetting the bed.
2. Your child will wake **as** they are wetting the bed.
3. Later on your child will **wake** to the **full bladder message** and get out of bed to **go to the toilet**.

alarms

If you are not able to use the alarm now, **keep going with the Healthy Habits** and encourage your child to try sleeping **without night nappies** for a few nights about **every 4–6 weeks** to check for any improvement.

Please do not use the alarm if there are any **wee or poo problems** – check first with your **GP**, a children's doctor (Paediatrician) or a Physiotherapist.

Please **do not use nappies, pull-ups,** regular **pyjama pants** or **undies** while using the **mat and bell** alarm – a pyjama top and silky boxer shorts are OK (as the wee will run off the silky material).

Pull-ups, pyjama pants or undies will soak up the wee and **slow down** the alarm waking the child.

The alarm will work better if the child is able to **wake quickly** after wetting.

Pyjama pants or undies **are OK** to use with the **Personal Worn Body Alarm**.

alarms

THERE ARE 2 TYPES OF ALARM

AND THEY ARE USED AT NIGHT ONLY

1

MAT AND ALARM (pad and bell). This type is used around the world.
It was first used about 100 years ago and is more expensive.
It is very **loud** and the **most successful** in treating bedwetting.
Price: about $1600–$2000 (may be hired for a few dollars a week).

Silent Wakener (vibrating disc) connects to the alarm box.
A large disc (dinner-plate sized) that goes underneath your child's pillow.
Instead of the alarm ringing, the **disc vibrates** to wake your child when they wet the bed.
This is very helpful for children that are **afraid** of the alarm, **startle** easily,
have **special needs** or a **hearing loss**.
Price: about $240.

Remote Buzzer (extension lead) for alarm.
Connects the main alarm in child's bedroom to a separate small box (buzzer)
that sits near the parent's bed.
It is useful when the parent's bedroom is far away, as you will hear the alarm
at the same time as your child.
Price: about $165.

2

PERSONAL WORN BODY ALARM (PWBA)

This is small – **matchbox sized** – and clips to the **pyjama top**.
A **cord** connects to a small **sensor** – this clips to the child's **undies**, near where the wee comes out. The wee makes the alarm ring (much quieter than the big alarm).

This type of alarm (PWBA) is **better for older children**,
as it can be pesky to turn off and re-clip on the fresh undies.
It can be bought as a **cordless** alarm.
Some types will make a different sound each time the alarm rings –
up to 8 different sounds.

Some can **record your voice** to use instead of the alarm/bell sound.
(This works well for children with **anxiety**, **special needs** or those very **sensitive to noise**).
Price: $120–$200.

alarms

USING THE ALARM

Encourage your child to help when possible,
as you are working **as a team** to reach dry nights.

No night nappies or regular **pyjama pants** while using the **mat and bell** alarm – nightshirts/nighties and silky boxer shorts are OK.

This will help the alarm to ring quickly after the wee starts coming out and wets the rubber alarm mat.

(Pyjama pants are OK with the PWBA, as the clip/sensor attaches here).

Protect the mattress as you usually do, and cover with a bottom sheet.

Put the **rubber alarm mat** (the size of a safety bathmat) on the bed, about where your child's hips will be and cover with a thin cotton sheet.

A **cord** connects the mat to the **alarm** (a box about the size of a brick that holds the bell and the battery).

Put the alarm box on the bedside table or under the bed – far enough **away** that your child has to **get out of bed** to turn the alarm off.

Place/**cover the cord** so that **no-one will trip** over it during the night.

alarms

Have your child do a **wee before** they get ready for bed.

They might like to read, listen to music or chat for a while.

Just **before lights out**, encourage your child to do **another wee** and then turn the **alarm on**.

Help your child do a practise **turning the alarm off**, **every** night.

This will help the child's **brain** to remember what to do when the **alarm wakes them up** as they start to **wee**.

During the night, **every** time the **alarm rings** your child needs to **turn it off quickly** and **go to the toilet** to fully empty the bladder.
(Your child may be very sleepy and may need help to find the toilet!).

Be sure to **wipe** the mat **dry** before the child **turns the alarm back on**!

Put a **dry sheet** over the mat and make sure that **your child is dry** and comfortable.

If your child sleeps through the alarm, go in and **help your child to wake up** and to **turn off** the alarm, then go to the toilet.

Leave the alarm **turned off after 2** wettings.

2 times a night is enough to train the brain to listen to wee message

alarms

YOU WILL NEED ...

A chart or notepad, pencil, clock, rags to dry the mat, spare cotton top sheets for the mat, a basin or bucket to put all the wet stuff in and some spare boxer shorts for your child.

New alarms come with instructions, and some have their own charts, or you could **copy** and **use the Wee Chart** at the back of this book.

It will be helpful to **write some things down** each time the alarm rings

- **What time** of night does the alarm ring?
- What size is the wet patch?
- How **quickly** did your child wake to the alarm?

How to know when the alarm is working

- Your child **sleeps longer** at night before wetting the bed.
- The **wet** patch becomes **smaller**.
- The child is **faster** at turning off the alarm.
- The child may **sleep through** the night or **wake** at night **to use the toilet**.

In the morning, encourage your child to help (teamwork!) by taking the bucket of wet things to the laundry.

The parent/carer takes the rubber mat to the laundry – **wipe** well with a wet cloth (**water** only), **wipe dry** and place over a laundry rack to finish drying.

Please **put the alarm away** if visitors are coming or if your household is very busy.

The **average** time to reach dry nights using the alarm is **4–6 weeks**.

We are aiming for **14** dry nights in a row.

OVERLEARNING

Most programs (for bedwetting) encourage 'overlearning'

(a drink challenge) once your child has been dry for 14 nights in a row.

It will help to lessen the chance of a relapse.

Set the alarm as usual.

Give your child a **cup of water** at bedtime **just before lights out**.

This can be for **7–14 nights**.

Your child will

1. **Wet the bed**, turn off the alarm as usual and use the toilet. Please tell your child **this is all OK**!
2. **Wake** to use the toilet.
3. **Sleep** through the night.

alarms

WEANING OFF THE ALARM

After the '**overlearning**', try leaving the alarm set up but **turned off** for a few nights, then a few nights **without** the alarm – **before** returning it.

If **not dry by 12 weeks**, it is usually advised to **stop** using the alarm for a few months and then try again.
Continue with **Healthy Habits**. The alarm can be used again as needed.
Talk to your Nurse or GP if unsure.

WHERE TO GET AN ALARM
From a pharmacy, a Continence Nurse, a Children's Hospital, eBay,
a supplier (Ramsey Coote or Malem) or nightollie.com (private alarm hire and program).

PROGRAMS FOR CHILDREN THAT ARE BEDWETTING
'Google' search bedwetting alarms/programs in your city, state or country or ask your local GP (Doctor), Child Health Nurse or at your Community Health Centre.

relapse

A relapse is when your child has **used** the **alarm**, been **dry for a month** or more, and is now **wetting more than 1–2** times a **week**.

Have another look at the **Healthy Habits**. Has anything changed?

Has your child been **unwell, overtired** or is **not drinking well** at school?

Your child may need to use the alarm again straight away.

Refer to www.hospitalhealth.com.au Nocturnal Enuresis Resource Kit second edition.

If **not successful** in having dry nights, please **see the GP**, as your child may need a referral to a Paediatrician (children's doctor).

The **GP** may order some **tests** to check the wee (for any infection), and perhaps an ultrasound of the bladder (to check for any wee leftover after using the toilet).

The **GP** may suggest a trial of some prescription **medicine** for your child.

medicine

MEDICINE

Your GP may suggest trying some **prescription** medication to help with bedwetting or to treat a 'twitchy' bladder.

MINIRIN to help the body make less wee during the night.
The Minirin Melt or Wafer is easy to take, and there is better control of the amount of the medicine than with the tablet or nasal spray.
Your child will need support when using it, as **drinks need to be stopped** for **1 hour before** and **8 hours after** taking the medicine.

DITROPAN comes as a tablet used to calm a 'twitchy' bladder.
This will help the bladder to hold bigger wees, hold on longer, have less accidents at school and less wet beds.

Sometimes these **medicines** are used at the **same time** as the **alarm**, sometimes **alternating** with the alarm for about **3 months** each.
Always keep going with the **Healthy Habits**.

Ask for help if you have questions or you are finding something is difficult to do.

hints

BE KIND

Please do not punish your child for wetting the bed. They cannot help it!

Please do not 'lift' your child from sleep to go to the toilet. This may save some washing, but will not help the brain to 'listen' to the wee message and will not help the child learn to wake by themselves.

Please do not stop your child having a drink when they are thirsty.

Do stay calm and help your child to drink well, use the toilet, change pyjamas after wetting and to have a wash or shower in the morning after wetting the bed.

Do encourage your child to help put all the wet stuff in the laundry in the morning. Together you and your child are a team!

Do encourage your child to tell you when they need help.

things to tell

OTHER THINGS

TO TELL YOUR GP, NURSE OR OTHER HEALTH HELPER

Is your child **well**?
Has your child had any **problems** with allergies, anxiety or anything else?

How your child **sleeps**.
What your child **eats** and **drinks** (most of the time).

Any **wee or poo problems** (also any problems **using the toilet**).
Do the Wee and Poo **charts**, and take them with you to your appointment.

Is there anyone in the **family** who has had bladder, bowel or kidney **problems**?

Does your child have trouble getting enough **exercise**?
What is your child like? (Any **behaviour** problems?).

Ask for help with changing to more **Healthy Habits**, if this is hard to do alone.

wee

ABOUT WEE

Does your child do **lots of very small wees** every day? (eg 10–20).

Does your child **leak** wee on the way to, or after using the toilet?

Does your child **leak** wee after jumping, sneezing or coughing?

Does your child to **hold** onto the wee for hours,
or **cannot hold** the wee, and is always 'bursting' to go?
(Have another look at '**Using the Toilet**' first –
does your child need help to change any toilet habits?).

Is the wee dark, smelly, hurts when it comes out?
Try having an **extra** 2 drinks each day.
See the GP if it hurts when your child wees, there is no change, or you are worried.

How the wee comes out

In a strong, steady stream?

As a dribble or 'stops and starts'?

Squirts sideways?

poo

ABOUT POO

Does your child **hold on** to the poo – or only do poos at home?
Does your child ever have any sneaky/leaky poo?

Does it hurt to do a poo?
How does the poo come out?
Lumpy, runny or as a sausage?

What colour is it: yellow, green, or brown?

Is it really stinky, frothy, slimy, or with lots of farts?
Tell the GP if you think the poo is strange (see the Bristol Stool Chart).

Giving the Nurse, Physio or GP **lots of information** makes it **easier** for them to **help** your child.

topsy-turvy

WHEN LIFE IS TOPST-TURVY

Keep coming back to **check Healthy Habits** for all the family.

Especially **keep going** with having **6–8 cupfuls** of water a day, starting with **2 cupfuls at breakfast** time.

At the **end of each month** check if your child is still **drinking well** most of the time (and at school).

At the **end of each month** check a few more **wee measures** (perhaps 2 each day for 5 days). A good start is that most wees are over 150ml.

Now your child is set and ready for using the alarm, whenever it is a good time for you and the family.

1 in 5 children will become **dry at night** whilst you are waiting for an alarm, and having mostly **Healthy Habits**.

Others may **wet less**, or even start to **wake to use the toilet** at night!

Please always be kind and patient with your child – to help them feel better about themselves, and also to get the **best results** on the journey towards dry beds.

Wee Chart

USING THE WEE CHART

Measure all wees, or as many as you can.
2 days measuring is good, **4 days** is better!

Your child will need to wee into a container (eg old ice-cream container) then pour the wee into a laundry measuring jug.

Write on the chart the date, **time**,
how much wee (eg ½ cup? 160ml?)
and colour & smell.
After measuring, flush away the wee.

Please **take the chart** with you on your visit to the GP or Nurse.
Lots of information will make it easier for them to help your child.

More information about healthy wee and poo (bladder and bowel), charts, pamphlets and other resources can be found at www.continence.org.au.

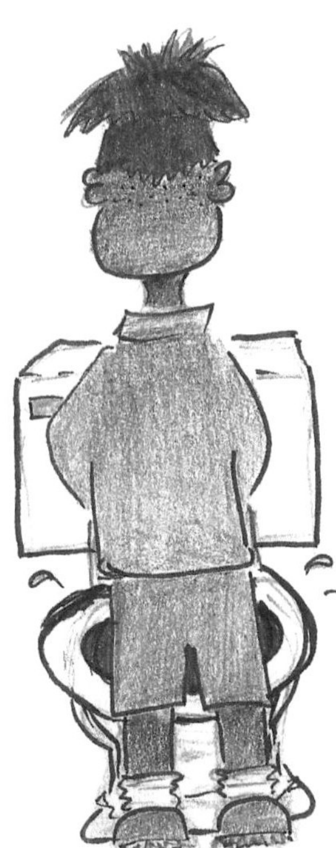

Please freely use, copy or photocopy this Wee Chart

WEE CHART

DATE	TIME	HOW MUCH	COLOUR & SMELL	WET PANTS

Measure wees for 2-4 days. Take the chart/s to the next appointment with your health professional.

Poo Chart

USING THE POO CHART

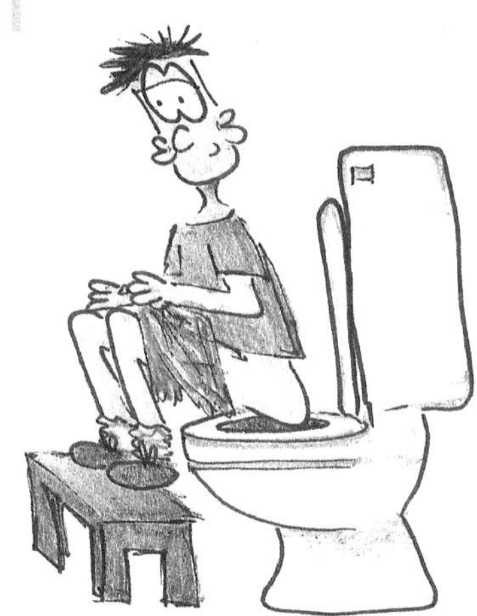

Look at all your child's poos (or as many as possible).
Ask them to call you **before** they flush it away!
(Just have a peek into the toilet bowl).

Write on the chart the date, **time**, **how much poo**, **colour & type and soiling**.
Using the chart for **7 days** is good, **14 days** is better.

Please take the chart with you to your visit to the GP or nurse.
Lots of information will make it easier for them to help your child.

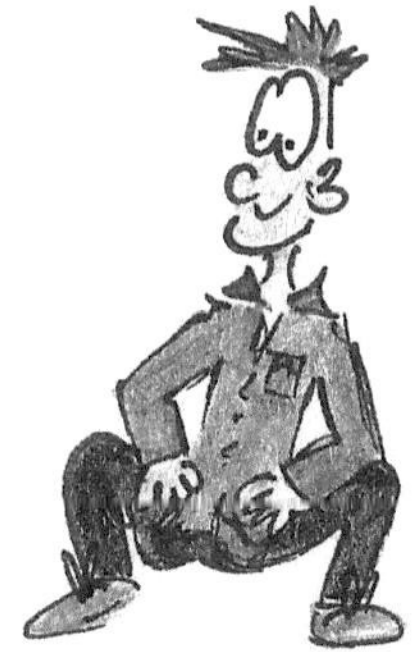

FOR POO TYPE
See **Bristol Stool Chart**
at www.continence.org.au

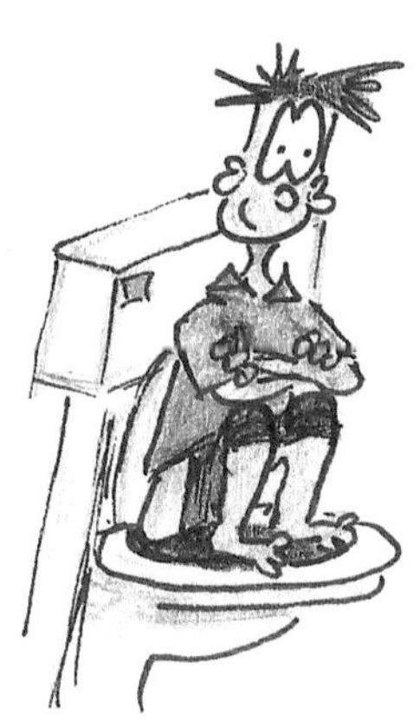

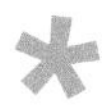

Please freely use, copy or photocopy this Poo Chart

POO CHART

DATE	TIME	HOW MUCH	COLOUR & SMELL	SOILING

Measure poos for 7-14 days. Take the chart/s to the next appointment with your health professional.

Drinks Chart

USING THE DRINKS CHART

Using this chart may help your child learn to **drink well** every day.

Every drink is a **cupful** – smaller cup for smaller children. **No more slurps**!
(Perhaps 150ml for a smaller child and 350ml for a teenager).

2 drinks to **start each day** (milk on breakfast cereal counts as a drink).
With a dry breakfast (like toast) a glass each of milk/water would work.

Encourage your child to **mark each drink** on the **chart**
with a ✔ ***or*** ☺ ***or some other marker.***
Have a chat at the end of each day – how did they go with drinks at school?
Your child may need an extra drink (always a cupful) on **a hot day** or **after sports**.

Encourage your child to **drink mostly water** and some milk.

Also try milkshakes; soy, almond, rice or oat milk (calcium enriched); fruit or herb tea; soup; homemade vegetable and fruit juice; watermelon, grapes and cucumbers.

For information on sugar in drinks go to www.who.int (nutrition)
and www.1health.gov.au

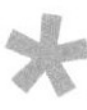

Please freely use, copy or photocopy this Drinks Chart

DRINKS CHART

	MON	TUES	WED	THURS	FRI	SAT	SUN
BREAKFAST	✔ ✔						
MORNING TEA							
LUNCH							
AFTERNOON TEA							
DINNER							

Have 2 drinks to start each day. Mark each drink with a ✔ or ☺ or some other marker.

resources

RESOURCES

Books

BOOKS FOR CHILDREN about wee and poo

Time to Pee Mo Willems, 2003
Potty Animals Hope Vestergaard, 2010
Funny Bums Dr Mark Norman, 2013
Everybody Poos Taro Gomi, 2012
Where's the Poop? Julie Markes, 2004
Poo at the Zoo Sarah Eason, 2011
The Story of the Little Mole Who Knew It Was None of His Business Werner Holzwarth & Wolf Erlbruch, 1994
Jurassic Poop Jacob Berkowitz, 2007
Who did that? Jill B. Bruce, 2004
Poo: A Natural History of the Unmentionable Nicola Davies, 2004
Pooflip Rob Wiltshire, 2018
What Bumosaur Is That? Andy Griffiths, 2007
The Fartionary Andy Jones, 2011

A great book about using the bedwetting alarm

Max Archer, Kid Detective: The Case of the Wet Bed Howard Bennett, 2011

About anxiety books for children

Slow Down, World Tai Snaith, 2017
All Birds Have Anxiety Kathy Hoopman, 2017
Hey, Warrior Karen Young, 2017

BOOKS FOR ADULTS

30 Days 30 Ways to Overcome Anxiety Bev Aisbett, 2018

Waking Up Dry Howard Bennett MD, FAAP, 2005 & 2015

Seven Steps to Nighttime Dryness Renee Mercer MSN, CPNP, 2004 & 2011

Getting to Dry Max Maizels MD, Diane Rosenbaum PhD & Barbara Keating RN, MS, 1999

It's Not Your Fault Joseph Barone MD, 2015

Websites

www.continence.org.au Bristol Stool (poo) Chart, pamphlets and booklets on wee and poo (bladder and bowel), and information about toileting children with special needs.

www.i-c-c-s.org International Children's Continence Society; membership, articles, conferences and resources

www.hospitalhealth.com.au Nocturnal Enuresis Resource Kit second edition (a brilliant training manual for health professionals)

www.eric.org.uk Information on bladder and bowel health

www.bladderbowel.gov.au

www.treatbedwetting.com.au Lots of information on bedwetting, checklist, an app for your phone and buy alarm

www.ramseycoote.com.au Buying and servicing of alarms (mat and bell)

www.nightollie.com.au Private program and alarm hire

www.thebedwettingshop.com.au Malem alarms (personal worn body alarm)

www.getmoving.tas.gov.au Exercise and activities for families

www.movewelleatwell.tas.gov.au Resources for nurses and teachers

www.dhhs.tas.gov.au Go to 'healthy kids'

www.who.int Go to 'nutrition' for information on sugar content in drinks

www.1health.gov.au Chart on sugar content in drinks

www.eatforhealth.gov.au Picture of healthy food plate

www.heartfoundation.org.au Healthy foods and great recipes

www.schn.health.nsw.gov.au>hospitals>chw Factsheets about good food choices

www.raisingchildren.net.au Good information on behaviour and development

THANK YOU

My mum, Glory, and my son, Nick, for all your love and support.

Jo, for giving this project momentum.

Kim, Hazel, Cindy, Christiane, Fiona and Robyn, for your valuable feedback and enthusiastic approval of this book.

Jenni, for your friendship and generous mentoring.

Ben, for your illustrations, bringing a lighter side to this sensitive topic.

Lucinda, for embracing my project with enthusiasm and a discerning eye.

Steve, for your abundant warmth and wisdom.

HIGH and DRY

ISBN 978-0-6486758-9-1

The charts contained in this book may be freely copied, photocopied or scanned.

Layout by Kent Whitmore

Published by Forty South Publishing Pty Ltd, Hobart, Tasmania fortysouth.com.au

Printed by RevolutionPrint revolutionprint.com.au

If you liked Ben's drawings in "HIGH and DRY" then you'll love

The Gods Must Be Disabled

GRAPHIC NOVELS BY BEN RICHARDSON

The first two books in a planned series culminating in Episode 1

A humorous look at members of a group with disabilities who are found to be old gods in disguise

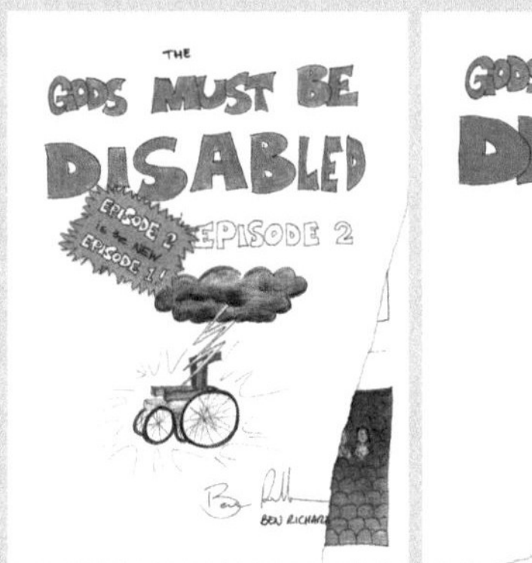

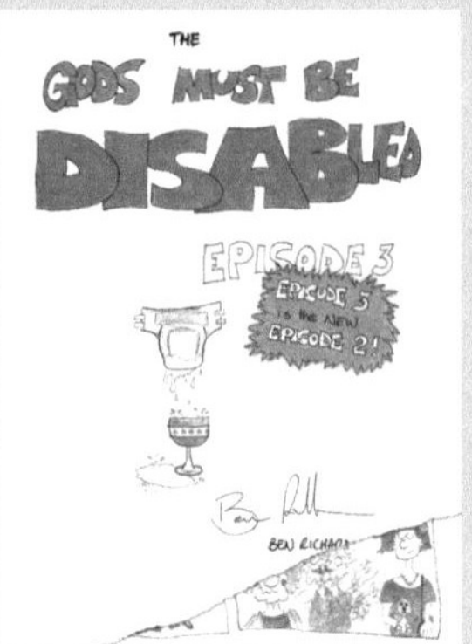

thegodsmustbedisabled@gmail.com

www.thegodsmustbedisabled.com

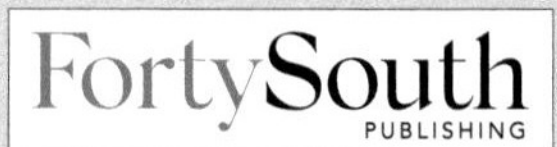

fortysouth.com.au

HUMOUR

$24.95 each plus postage

Paperback